W0232852

My Little Epiphanies

My Little Epiphanies

Aisha Chaudhary

B L O O M S B U R Y
NEW DELHI • LONDON • OXFORD • NEW YORK • SYDNEY

BLOOMSBURY INDIA
Bloomsbury Publishing India Pvt. Ltd
Second Floor, LSC Building No. 4, DDA Complex, Pocket C & 6 & 7,
Vasant Kunj New Delhi 110070

BLOOMSBURY, BLOOMSBURY INDIA and the Diana logo
are trademarks of Bloomsbury Publishing Plc

First published in India 2019

ISBN: 978-93-84898-20-5

6 8 10 9 7

Printed and bound in India

Bloomsbury Publishing Plc makes every effort to ensure that the papers
used in the manufacture of our books are natural, recyclable products made
from wood grown in well-managed forests. Our manufacturing processes
conform to the environmental regulations of the country of origin

To find out more about our authors and books visit www.bloomsbury.com
and sign up for our newsletters

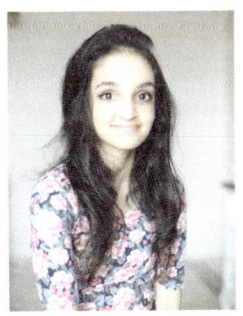

Author's Note

Before reading, I would like you to know that this isn't written like any ordinary book. It's more of a way to express my thoughts that come to me as the days go by. Actually, my days aren't very ordinary either. Not for an 18-year-old girl, that is. My name is Aisha. I was born with SCID (severe combined immune deficiency) and underwent a bone marrow transplant in the UK when I was six months old. I now live in New Delhi, India, where I was born. I have developed pulmonary fibrosis, which is a hardening of the lungs. I can't breathe, therefore, I spend each moment connected to an oxygen tank, and use a wheelchair while leaving the house as my heart cannot take it when I stand. Unfortunately, everyone has their problems and this is mine. I have felt isolated and completely stuck. So, I decided that it's time to reach out. I wanted to share my thoughts with the world. I wanted to let people know that they are not alone and, regardless of what the problem is, we all feel the same, and we are all fighting our own battles together. This book is about finding myself, letting go and expressing who I am, and I do hope that by the end of the book, you will find a piece of yourself too.

Dedication

Dear Tanya,

I'd like this book to be in honour of you. You are one of the many reasons I live today. If it weren't for you, I wouldn't be writing this. We went through the same thing, but you left the world as a baby. You will live in our hearts forever. I want to live tomorrow for us too. Sometimes, I look up at the sky and smile and feel you smiling down at me. I have never known you but have always loved you, my sweet sister.

I'll meet you in the skies, my angel.

Love,
Aisha

My dearest darling, Rolo,

I am just lost for words. I don't know how to breathe without you, my baby. You were the light of my life, you were one of the main reasons I forced myself to wake up every morning. You were my strength. You were my everything. You always took my illness upon yourself. I just wish you didn't take it this far. You left me so suddenly, but I have to remind myself that bad things happen for good reasons. You went to heaven at 8:30 AM on 2 December 2014, the day after Tanya's birthday. I like to believe that God gave you to her, as her birthday present. She probably needs you more than I do, my sweetheart. I know you are in good hands and are probably licking her face nonstop right now, as you once did mine. I imagine that she knows by now that you always yawn if she itches your cheeks, just like I once did. You brought so much happiness into my life; you were the sassiest pug I had ever come across and I just have to be grateful that I got to know and love you. You were the magic in my heart and you always will be. I will never forget you, 'Rolito, the Burrito'. Tanya and I shared the same disease and now we will share you too. You are her angel now. Look after each other. I will love you forever.

Sweet dreams, my precious.

Love,
Aisha

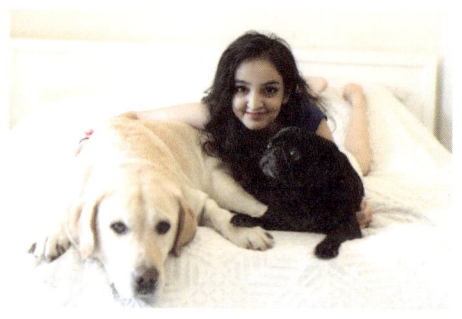

Fairy dust in your eyes
I could see no more
They say the soul never dies
What did yours leave me for
My darling you have kept me alive
You soothed the rocky roads before me
I'm shattered now you're dead inside
Burnt into thin air, this was our destiny.
Until we meet again, one day our worlds will collide.
Till then you always own a piece of my heart
Just tell Him not to further break it apart.

Foreword

Even though we never met, I instantly fell in love with Aisha Chaudhary through her story and the memories of those who knew her.

It's what motivated me to accept the role of her mother, Aditi, and to also co-produce the Hindi film adaptation of her life's story. And what a story it is!

You get an insight into that life with *My Little Epiphanies*. Authored by Aisha, this book takes us through every emotion—from hope, happiness and love to sadness, despair and loneliness—through her words and beautiful doodles. What she calls little epiphanies are actually life lessons, at least for me. I know it's hard to imagine taking advice from an 18-year-old girl, but then this was no ordinary 18-year-old girl.

It's the kind of book that makes you feel inspired and yet heartbroken. Many will feel her pain like it's their own and some may find solace in knowing that they are not alone in the various challenges that life throws. No matter how you feel, it will make you step back, look at everything you've got going for you and appreciate and enjoy the gift of life you have.

Through the book, you understand that we all go through a roller coaster of emotions every single day, but we need to find the courage to face the difficulties in life. You can't change the cards you've been dealt with... but the hand you play, that's on you.

I know what it's like to lose a loved one. You lose a little part of you with them, something that will never come back and all you have is a memory etched in your heart forever. Aisha has left that memory not just for her family but for the world through this book.

In the words of Aisha, 'Let's live and love with no regrets.'

—Priyanka Chopra

Prologue

My Dearest Darling Aisha,

I can never forget that day when I went to pick you up from school—you were only 12 years old and studying at the American Embassy School, New Delhi. In the car, I told you that a journalist had contacted me to ask about the circumstances surrounding our decision to have you, even though we knew you may be born with a genetic illness.

The Nikita Mehta Case was in the news at the time and we had been watching it unfold with great interest. I remember settling inside the quilts and animatedly discussing our feelings about a mother who was 28 weeks pregnant and who had moved the Mumbai High Court to request that she be allowed to abort her baby as doctors believed that he may be born with a heart condition.

Thankfully, I had always told you the truth about life and death so we could be very open with each other. Aish, you always take it all on the chin and I am in awe of your strength. Do you remember the time my friend was over at our home and I was talking to her about Tanya, and you, all of five years old, just ran up to us and said excitedly, 'You know I had a sister named Tanya and she died!' Then, you ran back, leaving my friend totally aghast! I think she had trouble falling asleep for a whole month!

I remember telling you, in the car, that since I had just started working at a drug and alcohol rehabilitation centre as a mental health therapist, I needed to lie low so I had refused the interview. I also recall saying, 'I like my privacy.'

But, you turned around and replied, 'Oh my God Mum, you are such a hypocrite! You keep reading true stories and telling me how much you learn from them and then you refuse to talk about your own life!'

I was so taken aback by how articulate and how 'right' you were. I had told you, *'Tu itna bolti hai… tu de de na* interview?' ('You speak so much… why don't you give the interview?')

And that's exactly what you did, that too on the Times Now channel at the age of 12 years! The reporter kept saying, 'Please go over the answers with her.' We were both appalled!

Needless to say, I insisted we hide your identity and you humoured me with that.

Fast forward to 2014, you loved the trailer of *Margarita with a Straw*; I think you could relate to the girl in a wheelchair. You were waiting for the movie to be released and kept asking me if you would be able to see it. Dad tried for many hours to find it on some online channel; meanwhile, we would just watch the trailer over and over again.

As you know, I saw the movie on Nani's birthday. I wanted to organise something meaningful for her as it was in April and you had left us in January. I decided to book tickets for *Margarita with a Straw*. I really wanted to go but I was scared witless. From 2010, we would do a high-five every time our plane landed in a new location, but all we did in 2014 was a high-five whenever we made it to the cinema hall to watch a movie. Movies were 'our thing'; we would watch one and then discuss it all to death. You know Aisha, even now, whenever I'm watching something, I instinctively turn to exchange a look with you... we always knew what the other was thinking, didn't we!

So, I was scared to see *Margarita with a Straw*, but then I recalled something you used to say, '*Darti hai? Chal ja kar ab!*' Your powerful message of 'be scared, but do it anyway... make sure to do the things that really scare you'.

Well, I went and saw it without you and in some way for you.

It is a hard-hitting, fabulous film which forces you to think but, how much I missed you, my advisor of all things Bollywood!

Then, Dad and I met a filmmaker in Mumbai; we were there for Dad's music show at the Hard Rock Cafe. The filmmaker was very keen about taking the story of your life to celluloid; I was taken aback and caught off guard.

I spoke about this to your friend Dia Mirza, who told me that a life, a story is nothing if it isn't told.

Her words stayed with me.

I still remember when Dia met us at a lung support meeting in Delhi at the Fortis Hospital. I could see that she was doing everything she could to keep you amused and entertained while you were in bed, unwell. And, when Dia showed you the recording of a new song over Skype, I overheard you telling a friend, 'I spent the day listening to the recording of an unreleased Bollywood song, what did you do today?' I love how sassy you are, my sass queen!

Anyway, later that year, in November, I called Virginia Holmes (remember how she was introduced to us via a common friend, that is, my crazy, fun-loving Ritu Pahwa and her friend Bijon Das? As you know, Virginia has a make-up school called Fatmu and had come to Mumbai with Danny Boyle's team for *Slumdog Millionaire*. She is a fabulous make-up artist but more importantly, she is British with an Indian soul). We still speak often Aisha, mostly because I love Virginia and feel very connected to you whenever I interact with her. After you left, Virginia sent me the poems you wrote together—the ones where you wrote one line and Virginia the next. They are beautiful.

I told Virginia about all these events and, on an impulse, I asked, 'Do you know any filmmaker I can run all of this by?'

As fate would have it, Virginia had done the make-up for *Margarita with a Straw* and arranged a Skype call with the director of that movie, Shonali Bose.

The Skype call was booked for 15 minutes but it turned into a 3-hour chat between two mothers who had lost their children in painful ways. I ended up asking Shonali if she would consider writing your story.

The next day, I woke up to an email from Shonali saying that she would consider writing the story but she also said that she went to her special place where she connects with her son Ishan and had the idea that there should be a documentary as well.

The more I thought about it, the more I realised that actually, Shonali was THE perfect person to tell your story—you loved the trailer of her film and left without seeing it; Shonali is very tiny like you (she even fits in your clothes!); she is both Indian and western in her outlook; she is a mother who has lost her child tragically and she is someone who understands the depths of pain and despair; like you, despite the challenges of her life, she has seized the 'bull of life' with both her hands! It HAD to be Shonali and no one else.

It is the hardest thing to tell someone your deepest thoughts and trust that they will do justice and portray your children for who they are. I knew that in Shonali's hands, we were all safe.

Shonali introduced us to Nilesh Maniyar who co-directed *Margarita with a Straw;* he has worked beautifully on your film as well. Aisha, thank you for leaving the name of your documentary in your poem—it's called *Black Sunshine, Baby!* Thank God, I remember how much you struggled, deciding between the two names for your book. Then, someone had said, 'Please keep the title, "Black Sunshine" because many people don't know what the word "epiphany" means.' The next morning, you told me you had chosen the title of the book to be *My Little Epiphanies.* When I asked how you had made the choice, you simply answered, 'If people don't know what the word "epiphany" means, it's good that it's in the title. It will give people a chance to look it up! After all, we read to learn, right?' Only you, my *gudia*, could think like that!

So now, Aisha, your film is selected in the Top 20 Gala Presentations at the Toronto International Film Festival. Why am I not surprised? You never did anything by half measures and I know if your name is attached to something, it's just going straight to the 'Pink Sky'!

Your documentary is well underway; I have seen glimpses and it's going to rock the world. I took what you said to me that day in the car seriously—I WILL give back, and in good measure, what I have learnt from living this life.

Did you hear the song Ishaan has made for you? It will be at the end of the movie. Ishaan calls it 'For Aisha' and you know it's the hardest thing for him to do. I am just so proud of him and his talent!

I will never understand how he got the music to flow like your life—sometimes up and sometimes down. I think he put your sassy attitude into it!

The song totally reflects who you are, and how you are. I can't believe he got it so right! *Achaa* now, don't roll your eyes!

Oh, I forgot! I was asked to write this because the readers will want to know how and why this movie was made! *Ab tu bolegi, 'Chal bak bak bandh kar aur kaam kar!'* ('Now you will say, stop your rambling and start working!') So, here it is...

This film was made

—because you said to Dad, 'I don't want to die' and now he is hell-bent on keeping you alive in any way possible. We believe that you live a little every time someone reads this book or gets to know or see you!

—because Shonali Bose had something to say about life and death and she JUST KEPT

GOING!

—because Siddharth Roy Kapur is a gentle, wonderful, smart and kind human being, and he and his team had immense patience with me!

—because Priyanka Chopra loved your story and is a gutsy woman, who is prepared to play a mother in the prime of her career!

—because you lived!

Because I love you so much!

I'll be with you in the skies one day my darling!

—**Moose**

Introduction

Me and Aisha

My darling child,

I have never met you. But, I feel I am totally inside your skin. If we had met, maybe this movie would not have been made. Maybe it was best that I made it from my imagination of you... Because a fictional film could never ever really capture you, and I might have given up trying! So it's good in a way that Fate kept us apart. In 2010, when my son Ishan died, one of your father's close friends (Bann Roy) called him from LA and told him he was shattered that his friend had lost her son. I was told much later that you were sitting right there and heard about what had happened. I love that you knew about my Ishan. Then a year later, I decided to move back to Delhi and we were trying to join the American School for my younger son, Vivan. Had he joined, I would have met you but, he didn't join and we didn't meet. And then, when I was making my film—*Margarita with a Straw*— my make-up designer, Virginia Holmes, taught you make-up and you ended up becoming friends. But even that did not lead to our meeting, and not even when you asked to watch my film. Your parents didn't realise then that there were quite a few people who knew us mutually and I would have definitely shown you the film. That film was *Margarita with a Straw*. We had had our world premiere at the Toronto International Film Festival (TIFF), just as *The Sky is Pink* will have too.

What I love most is that you watched the trailer of *Margarita with a Straw* 30 times and you told your mother that you hoped you live to see this film. You said that because, perhaps, you could feel the end drawing near. In fact, your body left Earth three weeks later. This was one of the first things your mother told me when she Skyped with me almost 10 months later. And then, she just blurted—would I make a film about you? She asked me not only because you had loved my trailer and both your parents loved my film, but because I too had lost a child. I said I would think about it.

Soon, she mailed me a copy of your book.

I think right from that moment you guided me! I read each of your epiphanies and I read between them as well. I SAW you and I honestly didn't think that you were a kid who wanted to be put on a pedestal as 'The Heroic Dying Teenager'. I felt that really strongly. If truth be told, I, myself, wasn't interested as a filmmaker to tell that story. For me, the interesting story was about the parents who went through this and whose marriage survived. Only the people who lose a child know that it actually alienates couples from each other rather than drawing them closer. I felt so guilty about ending my own marriage immediately after the death of my son that I researched this! I came across a book in the US where out of 50 couples (most of them happily married) who had lost a child, 45 ended their marriages. I found it fascinating that your parents didn't, and that they had met and fallen in love at the age of 16! This was the story I wanted to tell—the love story of your parents.

My next task was to convince them. You know how they are! So you know that it wasn't easy! They were hell-bent on a movie about YOU! Then, I came up with this idea (brilliant, if I say so myself) that they make a documentary about you. I asked my creative partner, Nilesh Maniyar, if he would direct this. I'm so happy he agreed. Thanks to you actually. He had read your epiphany—'Black Sunshine, Baby'—and was bowled over. That documentary is going to be absolutely brilliant and moving. I know he intends to bring you out as the artist that you were.

I've hijacked him for the last year to work on the fiction film which has delayed the finishing of the documentary. He has been integral to *The Sky is Pink* and I just couldn't spare him. In a way, the timing is perfect for the documentary to come out after the movie as people will want to know the real you. That's the end result but it was motivated by me (just between you and me!) to get your Mum and Dad off my back and let me make the film I wanted to!

I was living in LA again when all this about the movie and the documentary happened. I made a special trip to Delhi to meet your parents and hear their story. Your mother, as you know, has a photographic memory and can tell a story really well. She can also talk the hind legs off a donkey, especially if the subject is you! Nilesh and I went through two exhausting weeks of many hours just recording her. We heard about their lives from her childhood up until your death—52 years!

During that same trip, I mentioned to them about my philosophy of 'deathdays'. They are like birthdays but need to be celebrated and not mourned. I have celebrated every single deathday of Ishan—just as I celebrated, and still celebrate, his birthdays. The idea clearly appealed to them because the very next thing I knew was that your parents had converted your Dad's annual band performance with his Delhi University band into your *barsi*. In 48 hours, they had invited all their friends and relatives and there we all were in this beautiful club called Q'la in the Qutub area—celebrating you.

Before we left your house, I lay on your bed by myself. I closed my eyes and I felt your presence strongly (by the way, we would always do the recordings in your room, which is exactly the same as it was before. I love the energy in the room, it is utterly peaceful. Your mother loves it too). It was a cold night and your mother opened your cupboard—where all your clothes were still intact—and gifted me your short black woollen jacket. She said it was the first thing of yours that she was able to give away. I was deeply touched. Putting it on, I literally felt I was in your skin. At the *barsi,* I was amazed to see that how many people who were in your lives were in mine too! And still, we had never met. I had never even heard about you guys! There was Lushin Dubey who acted in my film *Amu.* There was the owner of Q'la, Sharyue Verma, who was in Miranda House with me. There was my friend Geeta Mishra from Columbia University days. There was even my college boyfriend, Samir Kuckreja! All close friends of your parents just like Bann, but fate and the Universe had conspired…

Your mother had told me that your brother was quite against this film being made. I told her right there and then that if he refused I would not be willing to do it. I felt very connected to him even before I had met him. Maybe because his name is also Ishaan! What are the odds of that! It made me feel this story was meant for me to make. Ishaan feared that the film could be unfaithful to your memory and to you. His notion of Indian cinema was just Bollywood. He didn't love it as you did! I was having a screening of *Margarita with a Straw* in New York (where he now lives, as I'm sure you know) and I invited him for that. In the Q and A session, I talked about my relationship with death and my Ishan. We went out for coffee afterwards and he just wept in my arms. It was beautiful. We immediately bonded. I completely understood him and his fears and his pain. I have a surviving son too after all. Ishaan loved *Margarita with a Straw* and after having connected with me, gave the green light.

Whenever your mother's narration had something about him, my ears would prick up even more acutely. It is no wonder then that when I finished writing the very first draft, I gave it the title—*The Sky is Pink*. I'm not sure your mother ever told you that story? While you were still recovering from the surgery in the hospital, she had gone to the public phone to speak with little four-year-old Ishaan. He was with your grandparents and father in Delhi.

Ishaan was stammering and crying, 'Mamma, the sky is pink, isn't it? But, the teacher said it's blue, and punished me.' Your mother reassured him that the sky could be any colour he chooses it to be. When she hung up, she went to pieces completely. So much so that the nurse had to take her to the hospital psychiatrist. Her courage couldn't stand up to the thought that her one normal child could be hurt in any way or that he had started stammering. I was deeply moved by this story.

I started writing the first draft of the script on your first deathday—24 January 2016. I breathed you in deeply and then just started writing. Almost immediately, the thought popped in my head that there should be a narrator and that narrator should be you, you as a spirit. The script starts with you narrating and I called you 'Spirit Aisha', to distinguish you from 'Aisha'. Right away, your voice was irreverent and funny—whether you were talking about your parents or about death, in fact, especially about death. The very first draft had the lines—'Let me get this out of the way right now, I'm dead! Yup, get over it. It's not tragic. I'm quite happy being a spirit, thank you very much, floating in the love and abundance of the Universe (you do know, you'll get here one day, right?)'.

I just felt deep in my gut that this would be your approach—to be irreverent and funny but also slipping a bit of philosophy every now and then. Spirit Aisha was a smashing success, and the big reason this film got green-lit. You—the real Spirit Aisha—was weaving magic from up there, no doubt, in cahoots with my own guardian angel, Ishan!

I'm writing this on a flight from Delhi to Bombay. We are in the throes of finishing the film for TIFF and it's the only time I can get. I am looking out of the window at the fat fluffy clouds and I visualise both of you prancing from one to the other. Or rather you lying languidly on one, and Ishan hopping around excitedly.

In this journey of writing and making this film, I have adopted your family and they me! We have a special relationship tied by death. Ishaan has cried in front of me and with me several times. Niren and I can talk about anything under the sun, including you, in a very comfortable way. I know that I can turn to him any time and he will be there for me. And Aditi has been completely emotionally naked with me. It is because of her that this script is what it is. There were times she would call me howling from Delhi (when I was in LA) and tell me something she knew I would immediately understand, even more than her own close people because we were both Mamma's who had lost our babies. But interestingly, you don't have to be one to understand one. One of my favourite scenes to do with death in the film has been written not by me but by Nilesh. It's a scene in which your mother is just sitting at your grave and cleaning it, methodically and calmly, like it's just a regular routine. She has a bag of cleaning supplies she carries with her and even shears to cut the weeds. Though Aditi has not specifically done this, Nilesh knew that she was very attached to your grave. She designed an absolutely stunning headstone for it. It took her a long time and she was really stressed about it as she's a perfectionist. I am sure you love it. We have replicated it completely for the film.

I know you're watching over your family. I want you to know I'm watching over them too. And I'll always have their back, especially Ishaan's.

I know you'll love one other thing that I did and that is to bring your sister Tanya into the limelight. This was something I divined, something that was not really told to me. I heard about her death from your parents, of course, but what I realised was that she was a buried source of pain whereas you were very much present. In making a film about you, I made her the centre, in a way. There was a scene that I had to take out of the film in which you cry to your mother and ask her if they will forget you too the way they forgot Tanya. Your mother replies that they have never forgotten her. Then, you say, 'But, why aren't there any photographs of her?' Your mother doesn't reply but we find out that it's actually because your father couldn't bear to have her photographs around and be reminded of her. Bringing out Tanya was my gift to your family and Aditi is very grateful to me for it. This was a real conversation you both had and it was acted out so beautifully by Zaira (a brilliant casting coup by Nilesh).

Your Mum said you would surely be smiling in Heaven to know that Zaira Wasim is playing you.

I was lucky that when my Ishan died, I was able to completely understand and accept it. He had spoken to me and told me, 'Mamma, I didn't have to be on Earth any more.' That made me realise that it's okay to die young. You're just a more evolved spirit, and from that perspective, your Tanu *didi* was an extremely evolved one. I know you have shown signs to your family too. I didn't really have any such belief system till Ishan died and connected with me... not like a ghost or a spirit talking literally, but deep in my heart; our feelings were so connected that death couldn't come in the way of that bond. I have read a lot about what might happen after we leave our bodies. I don't know how much I really believe but it makes me happy to think of you kids just rollicking around in the Universe somewhere and watching over us at the same time, staying with us in every single way except in the flesh. Maybe, you guys are really having a party in the sky, in the 'Pink Sky'.

Love you to bits,

Kisses and hugs.

Always,

Your

Moni (All my nieces and nephews call me that as I'm old-fashioned and I don't like my *bachchas* to call me by my name, and you're my *bachchi*.)

My Little Epiphanies

The fact that I'm sitting here, writing these words, is a miracle. I would not have been here, on this Earth, for more than a year had destiny not changed its mind.

We've all grown up, so why are we still playing the game of hide and seek?

Would the world be so bad if we were
all friends?

We all definitely have one thing in common,
and that is death.

What I'm going through is actually better
than what someone else is going through, out
there. But because we are so unaware and so
invested in our own lives, we can focus on
nothing but the shit; therefore, we will always
be extremely miserable human beings, no
matter what happens.

Life is a circle and we all think we are bang in
the middle of it.

She loved him but he did not love her and the stars were so perfect that night, but then, my darling, the darkness kicked in.

I hate myself for tripping into this beautiful thing everybody calls love.

I need a whole new pair of shoes. I'm running from myself this time.

I need to get over this and move on. It's making me too sad to enjoy my precious days on this planet. I can't give him the power to take that away from me too.

I crave the littlest things, while I've lost the biggest.

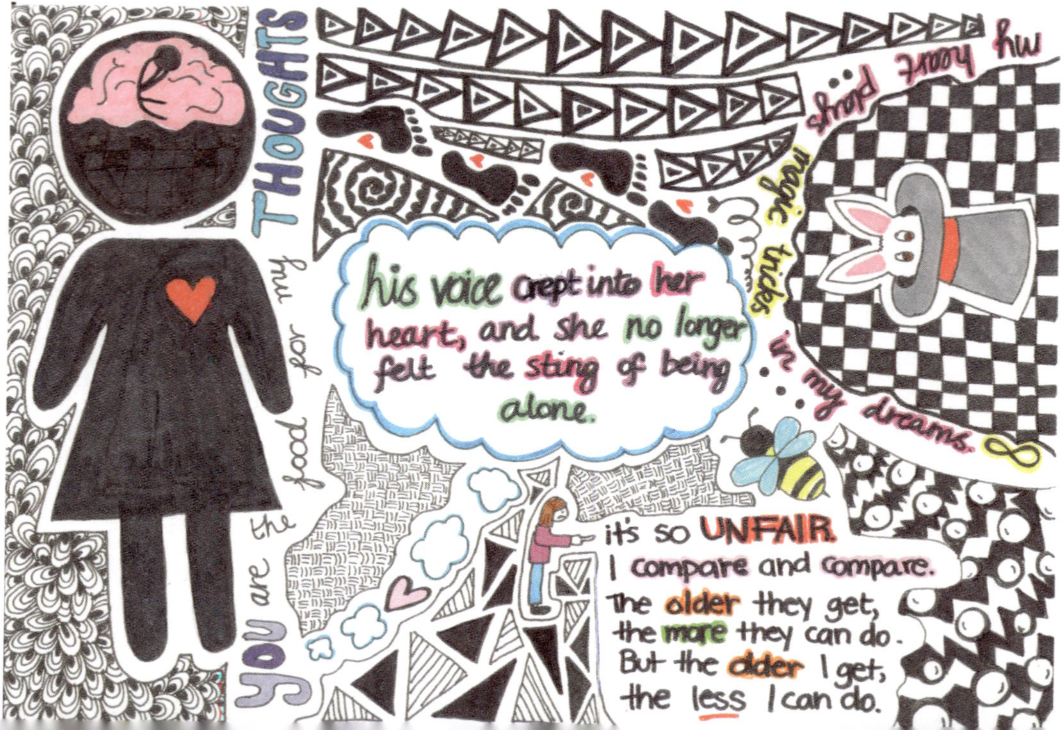
you are the food for my THOUGHTS
his voice crept into her heart, and she no longer felt the sting of being alone.
my heart plays magic tricks in my dreams.
it's so UNFAIR.
I compare and compare.
The older they get,
the more they can do.
But the older I get,
the less I can do.

Why do so many emotions exist?

This is everybody's problem—we keep looking up to find answers. Now, let's look within us.

Something must be wrong that even when the music is blasting, all you can hear is deafening silence.

When I'm high, it's like my soul is telling me a secret.

Death is a tricky business, and we are just the employees.

Are we living to die? Or are we dying to live? I
want to do the latter.

It's funny how we give each other blood in
order to survive. If we are willing to do that, I
don't understand how there is so much hate in
the world.

Don't worry about what happened today, death
is on its way—I promise you.

You're not my reality, you are just the reverse.

Heaven is not a place. Heaven is our home.

What is the definition of love?

A knot at the pit of my belly, a blessing and a curse. A gut-wrenching pain as though I've been stabbed; only instead of blood, butterflies disperse.

Do you ever see a stranger and think that they look exactly like someone from your past… only 10 years older?

Let's live and love with no regrets.

I can hear your heartbeats one after the other, like dancing rain on a dark, silent night.

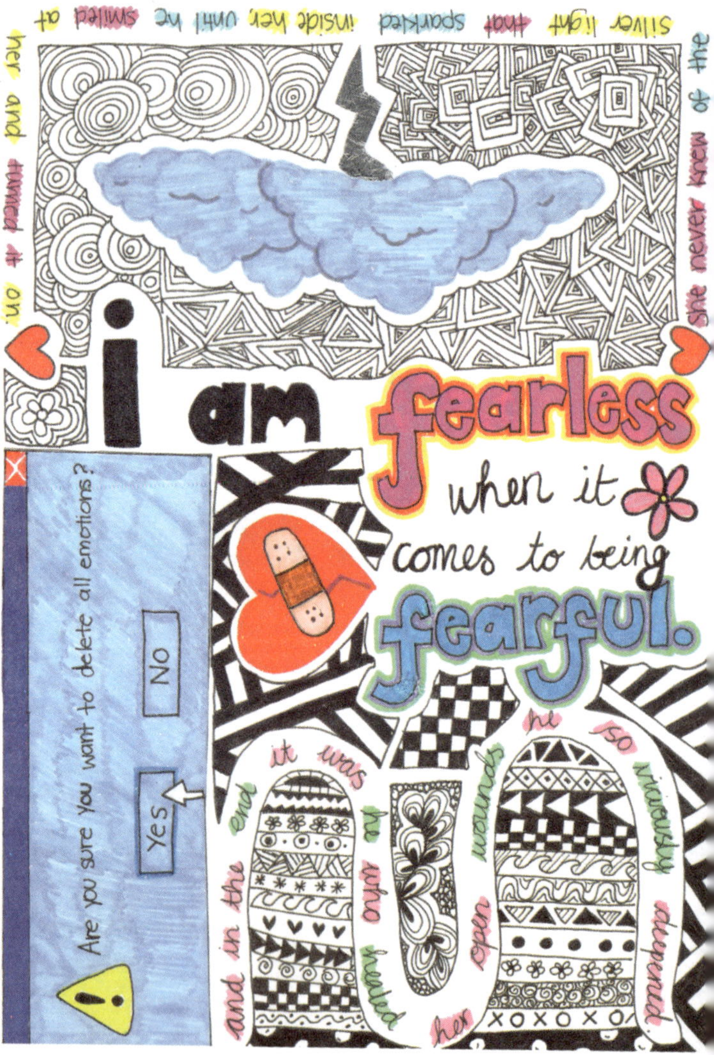
she never knew of the silver light that sparkled inside her, until he smiled at her and turned it on.
i am fearless when it comes to being fearful.
Are you sure you want to delete all emotions?
Yes
No
and in the end it was he who healed her open wounds he so viciously deepened.

My heart is tingling.

Mama says, 'Darling, if you have to go through shit, do it looking like a million bucks.'

Are we all fake at some level?

Shhh… miracles are happening.

Maybe in 10 years, you will be looking from the other side of the road and reminiscing about this time.

My mother must worry with every bone in her body.

It feels like I'm watching my world from above.

Let's wake up from this dream and turn it into a reality.

Thoughts come into your head 100 times faster, increasing exponentially.

We are the oldest we will ever be right now.

My lungs feel like ropes that have been tangled and knotted together, churning around in the pit of my belly, while my heart aches and cries in pain. Only, it's not the disease this time.

Being depressed just means that I'm
under repair.

If life is a stop at the station, I must admit I
don't want to get on the coming train.

I know there are healthy people out there who
feel as shitty as I do. But I don't know what
healthy is anymore; I'm stuck here, so how can
I really know about anybody else?

It has come to a point where I feel embarrassed
of my dreams.

In the end, overthinking is poison to
the heart.

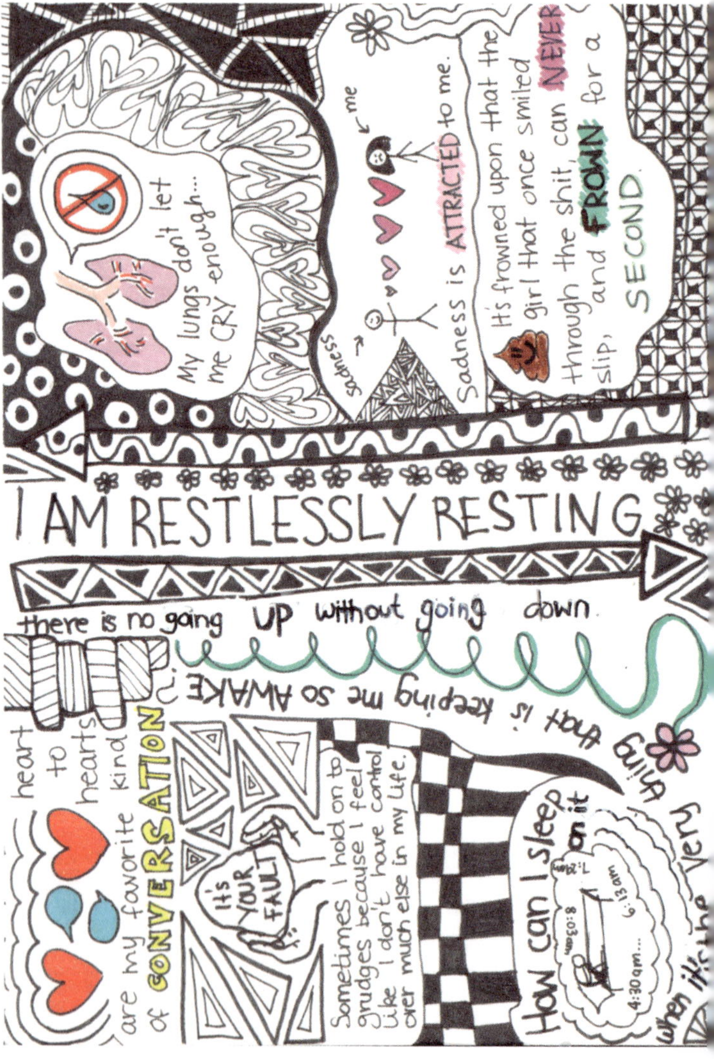

My lungs don't let me CRY enough...
sadness
me
Sadness is ATTRACTED to me.
It's frowned upon that the girl that once smiled through the shit, can NEVER slip, and FROWN for a SECOND.
I AM RESTLESSLY RESTING
there is no going UP without going down
heart to hearts kind are my favorite kind of CONVERSATION
It's YOUR FAULT
Sometimes I hold on to grudges because I feel like I don't have control over much else in my life.
How can I sleep on it
4:30 am...
6:13 am
7:29 am
8:03 am
when it's the very thing that is keeping me so AWAKE?

How is my heart functioning when it feels
so broken?

When your happiness starts to depend on
somebody else, protect yourself because you
are fucked.

I'm waiting for a surprise... that really defeats
the purpose, doesn't it?

I just saw things from his eyes and, in that
moment, my heart slipped away.

What is his soul making him think? Is it that I
am not worthy?

Maybe I am too real to be touched. Maybe
that's the problem.

What would happen if I wasn't in my own
shoes anymore? If I didn't have the life I'm
living this very second? What if I didn't know
the people I love so much today? What if I
didn't do the things that I love to do in this
moment? What if I wasn't all the qualities
which fill me with who I have become today?
What if I didn't feel the things I'm feeling as
I'm typing this word? What if I wasn't me?

I think we are the truest versions of ourselves
at night before we go to sleep, just before we
close our eyes.

There's only one type of fish in this sea and that is the selfish kind.

Other people's dreams are coming true, their memories are being created, their life is happening outside these four walls, and I am still here… I am still me.

If emotions are bags, I've gone so far through the sadness bag that I ripped a hole at the bottom of it.

They say you have to love yourself before you love someone else. But then again, they also don't like selfish people.

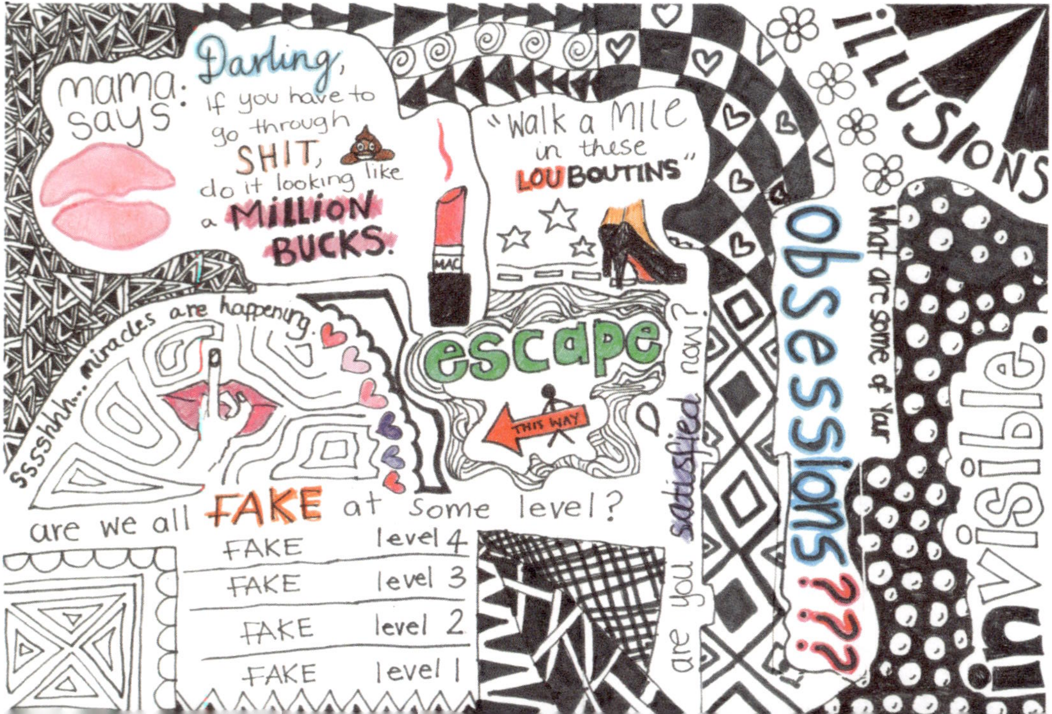
mama says:
Darling,
If you have to go through SHIT, do it looking like a MILLION BUCKS.
"Walk a Mile in these LOUBOUTINS"
MAC
escape
THIS WAY
ssssshhh... miracles are happening.
are we all FAKE at some level?
FAKE level 4
FAKE level 3
FAKE level 2
FAKE level 1
are you satisfied now?
What are some of Your
obsessions???
iLLUSIONS
invisible

D E A T H—Drop Everything And Trust Him.

I'm merely trying to survive until my respective death.

It's frowned upon that the girl who once smiled through shit can never slip and frown for a second.

I will do a cartwheel one day and on that day, I will say, 'I've made it.'

I want things to not be what they are, and what they are to not be.

Lie down, kick back and listen to the sound of
your heart falling in love.

They are watching me like I am some
TV show.

They say that there is such a thing as a
soulmate, but mine is the only one that will
die with me.

I had love for you, but lost respect for myself.

Why do we put those we love on a pedestal so
high that it's impossible to reach?

You know you're in love when their spark
ignites the light in you.

Even bad moments are moments, you know.

I want to get over you, but I want you to do
things, and when you do them, I love you.

If you feel like things aren't moving, there is a
cure for that, and that is time.

I feel like I have to keep reminding myself that
this is really just a phase and I'm going to get
over it.

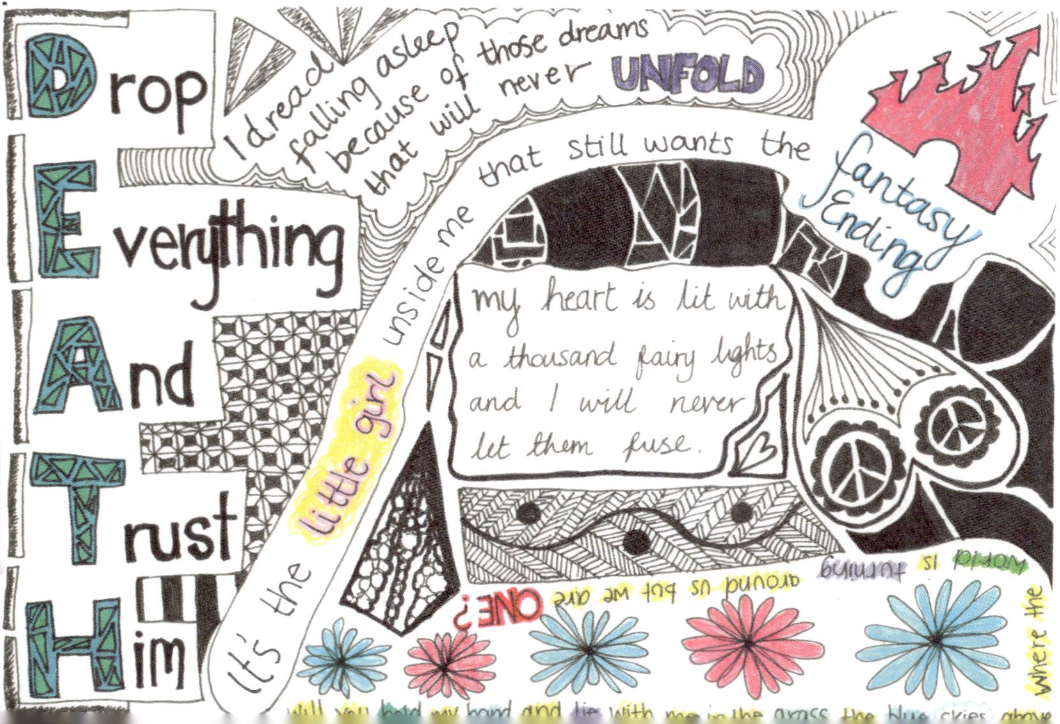

Drop
Everything
And
Trust
Him
I dread falling asleep because of those dreams that will never UNFOLD
It's the little girl inside me that still wants the fantasy Ending
my heart is lit with a thousand fairy lights and I will never let them fuse.
where the world is turning around us but we are ONE?
will you hold my hand and lie with me in the grass the blue skies above

I believe our little world is bigger and better
than the entire universe in some way.

If you could only know how loved you made
me feel that day.

People think I should be thrilled that it's not
yesterday, just because I'm better today.

These people who give me advice can breathe
for themselves, and I am just not applicable.

My body is sinking and I can't seem to find
which way is up.

I hope I'll never forget you in the hopes of
remembering.

Why is sadness so unattractive?

Sadness is attracted to me.

I am sad because I am sad.

I despise the feelings that come with jealousy.

I dream of the littlest moments I hope will
become my future. I dream of one of my aunts
asking at my wedding where is the one I'm
going to marry, and I whisper to her,
'Come, let us find him.'

What is living if I can't breathe?

You know you've won the game when the person who used to bully you and make life hell, recognises how far you've come and feels bad for their earlier doings.

I've forgotten what it's like to wake up in the morning without feeling the insides of my lungs.

It's the worst for me. I am suffering. It is my body that is broken.

If life is the show and we are the puppets, I wonder who is watching.

There is no going up without going down.

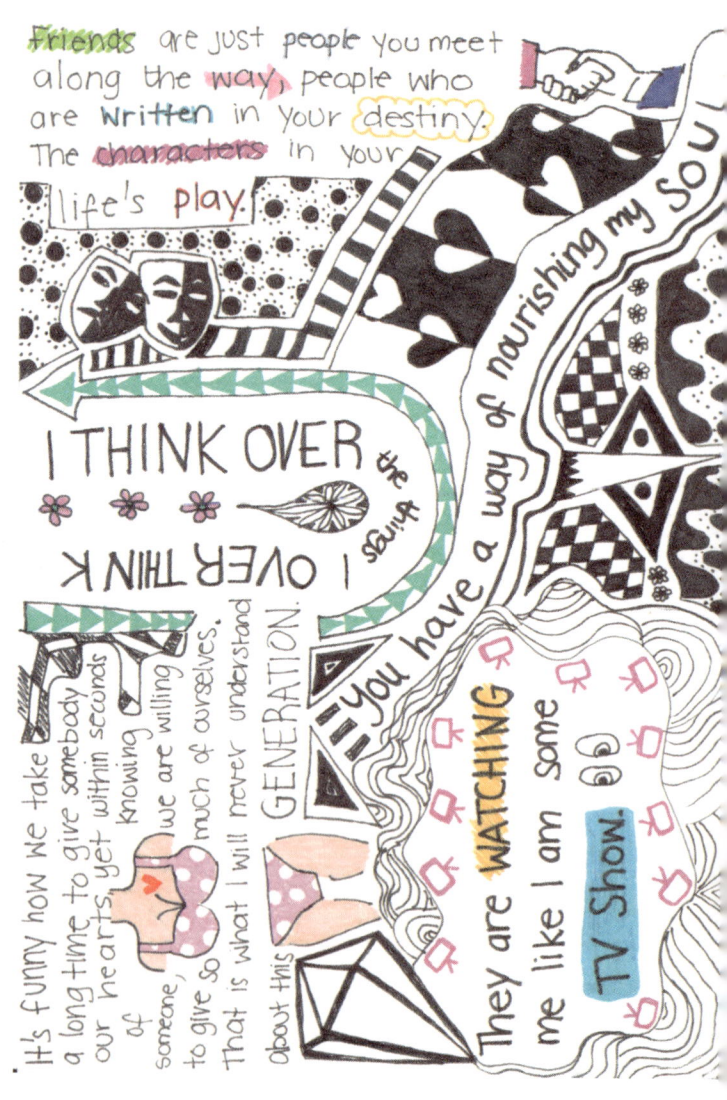

Friends are just people you meet along the way, people who are written in your destiny. The characters in your life's play.

nourishing my soul

I THINK OVER the things I OVER THINK

It's funny how we take a long time to give somebody our hearts, yet within seconds knowing we are willing to give so much of ourselves. That is what I will never understand about this GENERATION.

you have a way of

They are WATCHING me like I am some TV Show.

And in that moment I realised—if I keep him close, I fall deeper in love, and if I let him go, I will soon not remember. Which of the two makes me happier? That is the question.

Being bathed head to toe by someone else at 18 years old triggers insanity.

In the end, it's the little things that make us big.

It's funny how we take a long time to give somebody our hearts, yet within seconds of knowing someone, we are willing to give so much of ourselves. That's what I will never understand about this generation.

Heart to heart is my favourite kind of conversation. It is the way to feel the most connected to a person.

Your problems are my problems, and that is never the case.

The cure for any sadness is the connection with the people we love. Once you've lost all connection, then you know you're losing the battle.

I'm at a place so low that if anyone does anything in the slightest way to push my buttons, I become angrier than I actually should be... it's the scariest when it feels like you're out of control.

Having lost something so big has taught me to
appreciate the littlest things. I am blessed that I
have my eyes to see the vividness in the green
trees. I am blessed to have my sense of smell,
so I can inhale (pun intended) that particular
musty scent that hangs over Delhi after a day
of rain. I am blessed to have my ears, so I can
listen to the sound of my mother's laughter.
I am blessed to have my lips, so I can speak to
those I love. I am blessed to have my hands, so
I can paint whenever I please. I am blessed to
have my legs, so I can still walk on this Earth. I
must remember that I am blessed.

I'm going through this, therefore, I am real, but
what am I really real for?

To think that you don't love me is painfully
disappointing.

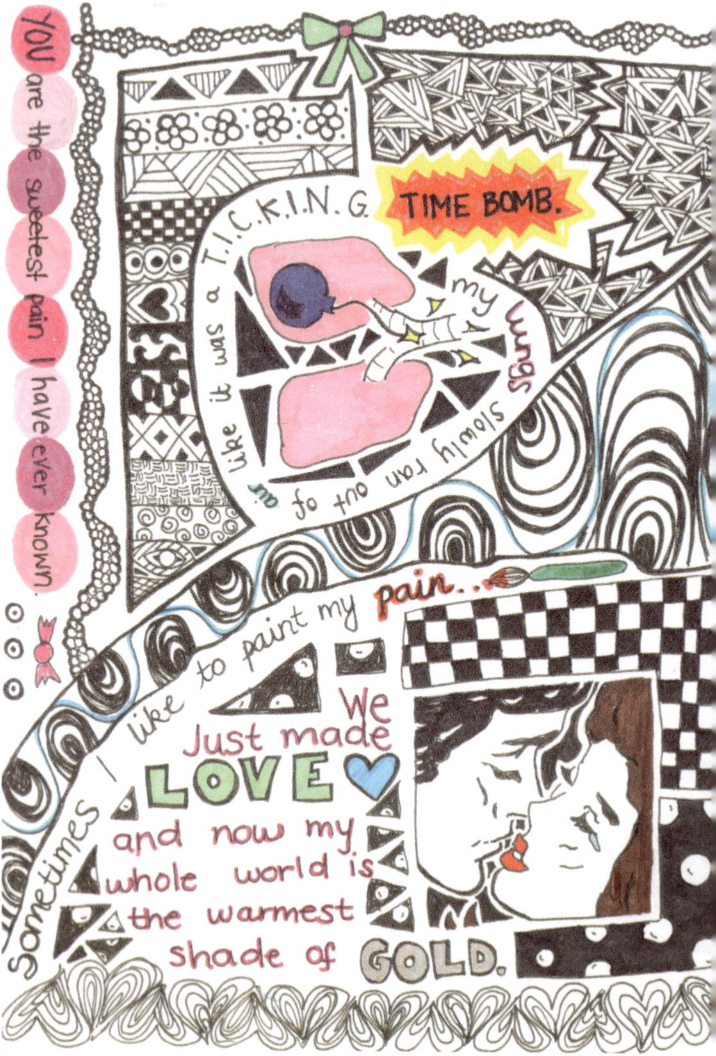
YOU are the sweetest pain I have ever known.
like it was a T.I.C.K.I.N.G TIME BOMB.
my lungs slowly ran out of air
Sometimes I like to paint my pain...
We Just made LOVE and now my whole world is the warmest shade of GOLD.

I really don't know what I know that I don't know.

I'm so stressed that falling asleep feels like a nightmare.

I think that we get really pissed at the superficial, irrelevant things, when we are really pissed at what our lives have turned into. I think that is the underlying truth.

I feel sorry for myself, and then I just tell myself, 'It's okay.'

Just being with a loved one is a real mood lifter.

I like to paint my pain.

I find that I do not remember the various invasive surgeries and trauma I went through as a baby, or even in the recent past. My mind has learnt to erase the pain I know I will want to forget, and for that, I am very grateful.

So let's succumb to the inevitable truth; death is upon us and we are all screwed.

It's weird how once we never knew the people we know now.

I'm hanging on for dear life, literally.

What is, is, and what will be will be, and what
never really was, was it?

My head is the room and my thoughts are the
elephants, and I am just so awkward.

Maybe sadness is unattractive, so we are
conditioned to want to feel it less.

Sometimes I hate myself and myself
hates me too.

If I look back on my early teen years, I realise
I had lungs but lacked self-confidence. Now I
have self-confidence but my lungs are lacking.
Which of the two is better?

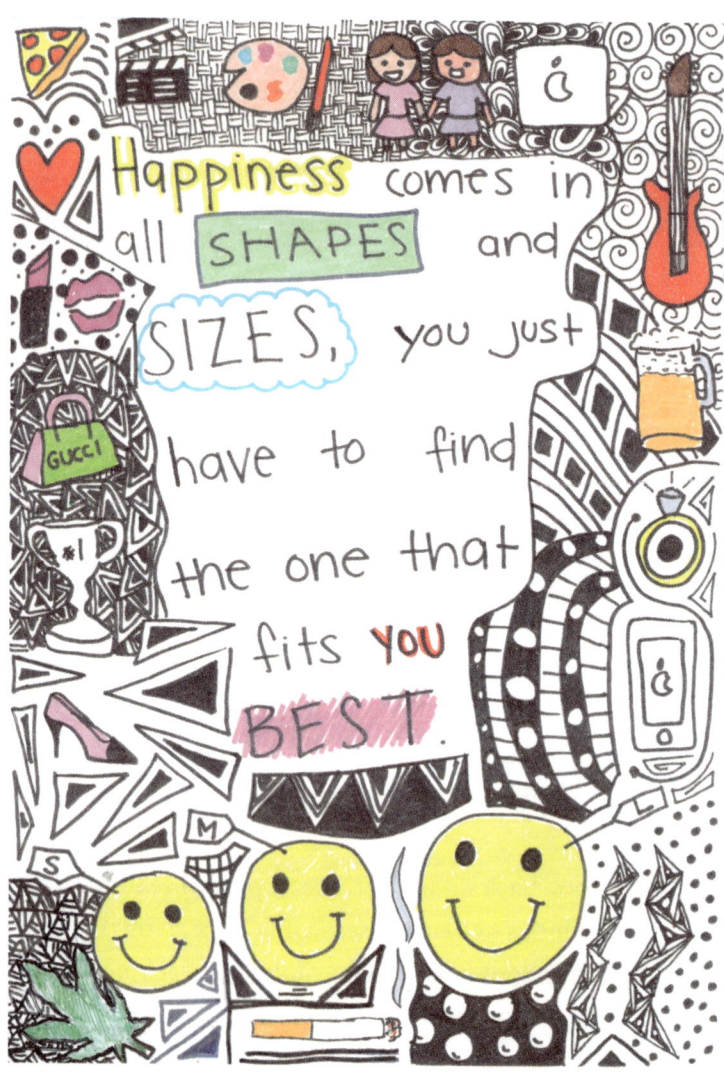

Happiness comes in all SHAPES and SIZES, you just have to find the one that fits YOU BEST.

It seems like everyone else is wearing a sugary coat and I am the only one wearing the salty kind.

It's like I'm being sucked in by quicksand, which is my disease.

Some words are worth gold. Say them while you still can. Say sorry. Say I forgive you. Say thank you. Say you are welcome. Say I love you. Say I love you too.

It's the scariest when I feel my own spark start to slip away from my own body.

Darkness has emerged into the light, and winter is coming.

My heart is lit with a thousand fairy lights. I will never let them fuse.

I must admit I am jealous of everybody I see. I see girls just standing up and chatting with one another. They look so healthy and I would kill to be them, and just be able to stand up too.

Let's swallow our feelings because saying how we truly feel is not really the done thing these days.

I don't want to be so transparent that you know exactly what I'm thinking, yet I don't want to come across as absolutely fake. Is there a place in between?

Self-recognition is the best kind.

I remember when I was little and it rained; I used to think that God was sad at the world and the rains were his tears.

Sometimes I find it easier not to talk or even put a smile on my face, and sometimes, I think that is okay.

If I was not like this, I would not have met the people I love so much today.

Happiness comes in all shapes and sizes; you just have to find the one that fits you best.

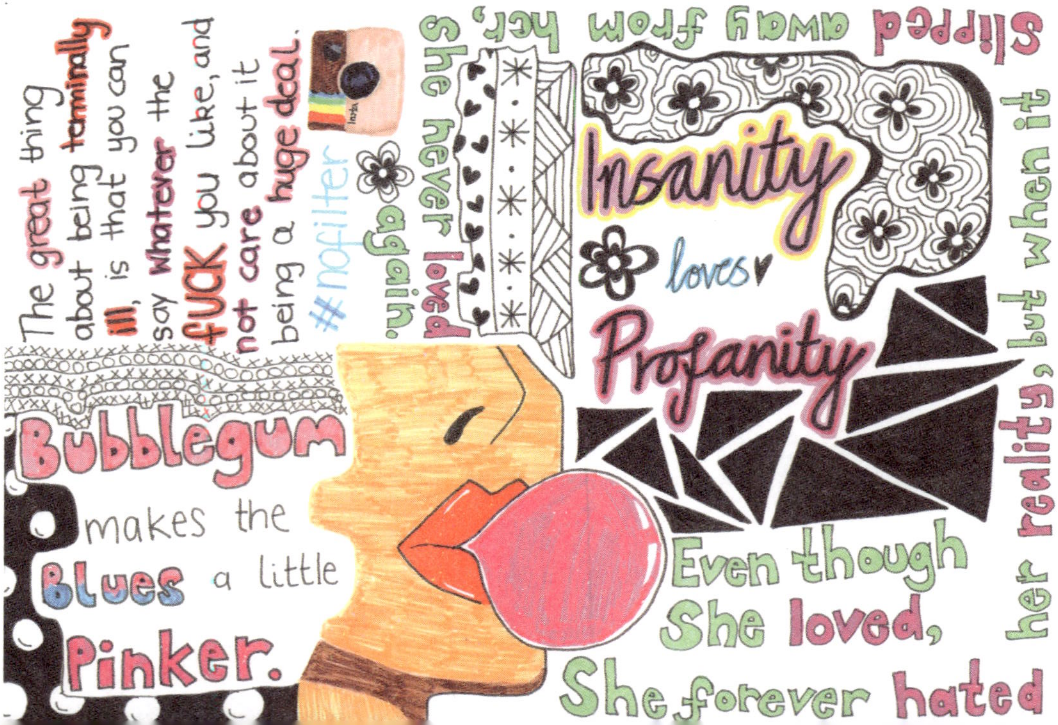
The great thing about being terminally ill, is that you can say whatever the FUCK you like, and not care about it being a huge deal.
#nofilter
Insta
Bubblegum makes the Blues a little Pinker.
Insanity loves Profanity
Even though She loved, She forever hated her reality, but when it Slipped away from her, she never loved again.

I do like the superficial things too. They allow me to decorate my body. Those things bring me to life, even when I don't feel very alive.

I am so weak; my only way to shout is to be strong.

I felt my lungs were steadily running out of air, like it was a ticking time bomb.

I don't want to jinx it, but I should be grateful that I haven't had three life-threatening diseases.

I want to make you see the world through the eyes of my soul.

Sometimes it makes me happier to hold on
to a grudge than to consider letting it go.
Holding on to it gives you a weird sense of
power and it almost feels like you have the
upper hand. It's my choice whether I fall into
that trap or not.

When I'm sad, people tend to brush it under
the carpet, but I can't do that because I am
the dirt.

My biggest fear of death is the notion that it is
all over.

The love I had for you was just another
bad influence.

I have come to accept the sadness within me.

It's funny how we all see common random
things in the day and connect them to our
own life's situations. We all see the same
news on TV, we see the same movies, read
the same books, but it means something
different to each of us. We look at things
from wherever we are in our lives and move
on from it thinking something entirely new.
Life is full of countless perspectives.

You have a way of nourishing my soul.

If I didn't have this life and I had that life, I would
still pine for another life that was not my own.

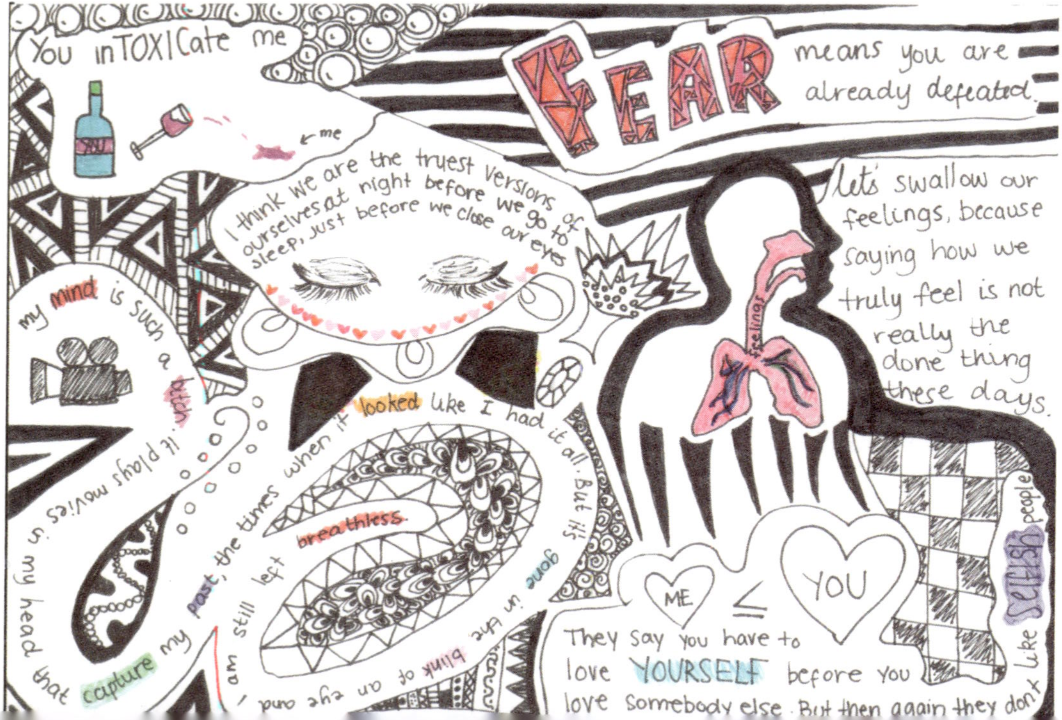

You inTOXICate me
YOU
← me
FEAR means you are already defeated.
I think we are the truest versions of ourselves at night before we go to sleep, just before we close our eyes
Let's swallow our feelings, because saying how we truly feel is not really the done thing these days.
feelings
my mind is such a bitch. It plays movies in my head that capture my past, the times when it looked like I had it all. But it's gone in the blink of an eye and I am still left breathless.
ME ≤ YOU
They say you have to love YOURSELF before you love somebody else. But then again they don't like SELFISH people

My thoughts have become my best friends, and
I really don't get along with them.

I think over the things I overthink.

It's the little girl inside me that still wants the
fantasy ending.

I want to live without being pitied.

If anything, it's wonderful to know that there
are people like you in this world.

A dramatic life calls for a little dramatic
thinking.

When I was younger, I used to think I was the
sickest I was ever going to be. Today, I still think
that, as I lie down with the oxygen tube in my
nose. What's around the corner? I don't ever
want to know.

We are in the most vulnerable state
when we think we are about to die. I think
we mostly get one main thought that gets
stuck in our hearts. It is either, 'I should
have said this' or 'I should have done that,
I should have been this'. If you are lucky
enough to get a second chance at life, you
must say it. Do it. Be it.

If you can't change your own life, there's
always someone else's.

How can I sleep on something when it is the
very thing that is keeping me awake?

I have come to accept the sadness that
overwhelms me.

The hard part about being determined is
staying committed and vice versa.

All our thoughts get recreated in the universe,
written down in God's plan for our future.

It's only now that I can almost see what my
body feels.

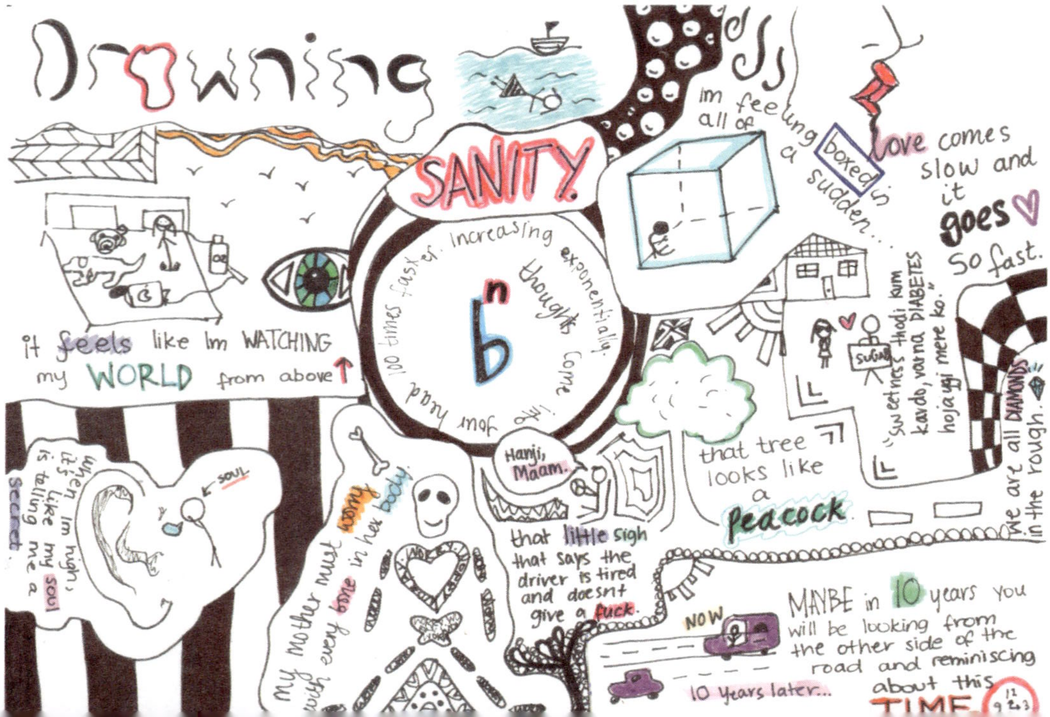

Drowning
SANITY.
b^n
100 times faster. increasing exponentially. thoughts come into your head
im feeling all of a sudden... boxed in
love comes slow and it goes so fast.
"sweetness thodi kum kardo, varna DIABETES hojayegi mere ko."
SUGAR
We are all DIAMONDS in the rough.
that tree looks like a peacock.
Hanji, Maam.
that little sigh that says the driver is tired and doesnt give a fuck.
MAYBE in 10 years you will be looking from the other side of the road and reminiscing about this TIME
NOW
10 years later...
it feels like Im WATCHING my WORLD from above
my mother must worry with every bone in her body.
SOUL
when Im high, it's like my soul is telling me a secret.

It's like I can already see things that are slowly being born into the truth.

I felt my feet stepping closer into the relationship.

Just because I was strong in one moment of weakness, doesn't mean that I am strong enough to be in each moment.

Things that are brushed under the carpet always have a way of getting stuck in our hearts forever.

Lovestruck by your presence upon me.

When you're unwell for a really long time, it becomes your identity.

Will you hold my hand and lie with me in the grass, the blue skies above, where the world is turning around us, but we are one?

I never thought about my lungs when they were healthy.

Pain lingers in the mind longer than it really lasts.

When I feel the monotony of my day turn into sheer pain, the only thing I can really do is stop and appreciate whatever I may be doing. Just stop and listen to the words in the movie I am watching. Just stop and feel the soft fur on my dogs and give them a million kisses. Just stop and embrace the hot water on my body in the shower. Just stop and look at my surroundings. Just stop and take in the sweet taste of my favourite candy. We should just stop for a second because one day, we may not be able to start again.

There is a lot of you in my heaven.

Sometimes the jealousy really gets in the way when I want to connect with someone.

Even when we are in a group setting and not saying something, something is always being said.

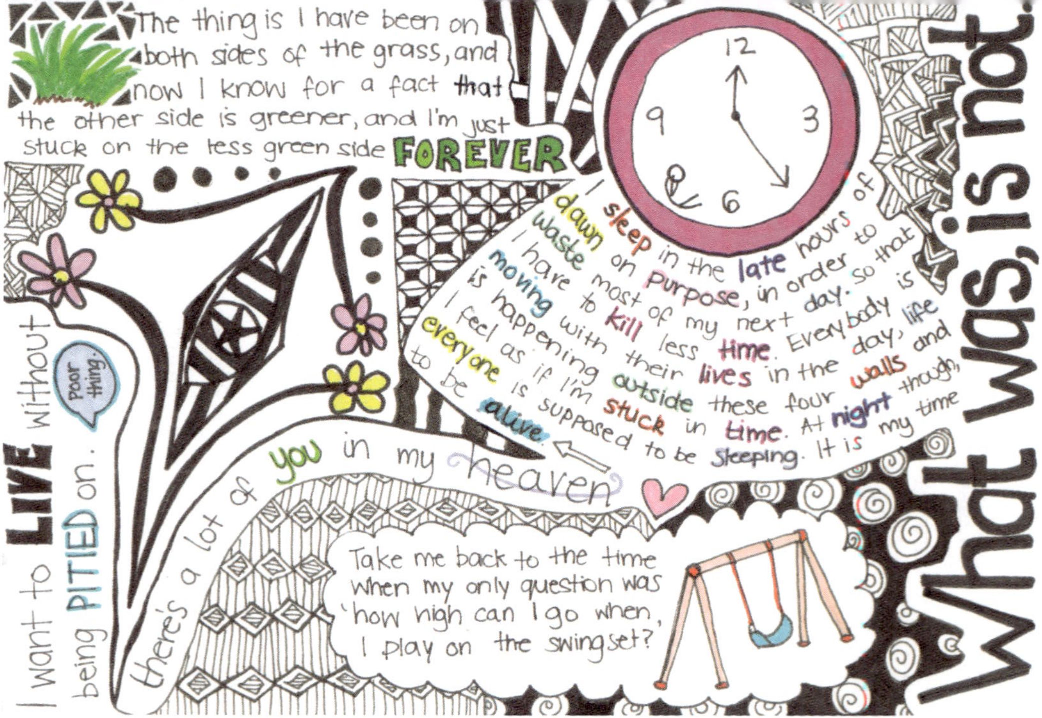

The thing is I have been on both sides of the grass, and now I know for a fact that the other side is greener, and I'm just stuck on the less green side FOREVER
12
3
6
9
I sleep in the late hours of
dawn
waste on purpose, in order to
I have most of my next day. So that
to kill less time. Everybody is
moving
is happening with their lives in the day, life
I feel as if I'm outside these four walls and
everyone is stuck in time. At night though,
to be alive is supposed to be sleeping. It is my time
I want to LIVE without being PITIED on.
Poor thing.
there's a lot of you in my heaven
Take me back to the time when my only question was 'how high can I go when, I play on the swingset?'
What was, is not.

It's heartbreaking to hear people talk about the future when your first thought is to wonder if you would still be around.

When is the right time to die?

Sometimes I hold on to grudges because I feel like I don't have control over much else in my life.

It's ironic because I want more time, yet I'm struggling to cope with a lot of it.

My lungs don't let me cry enough.

Even though I'm not okay, I must remember
that sometimes other people may not be okay
too.

Knowing all the facts doesn't make anything
easier.

I should be grateful that the shit isn't shittier
than what it's about to be.

I am restlessly resting.

The minute you realise you're thinking about
dying more than living is the moment you
need to change gears.

We are so selfish because we are never truly
in love with another human being. We are
just in love with a reflection of our desires, an
idealisation of a dream, which, in the end, is
merely our own.

I dread falling asleep because of those dreams
that will never unfold.

Has anyone else hit the bottom of this rock?

What was, is not.

Friends are just people you meet along the
way; people who are written in your destiny,
the characters in your life's play.

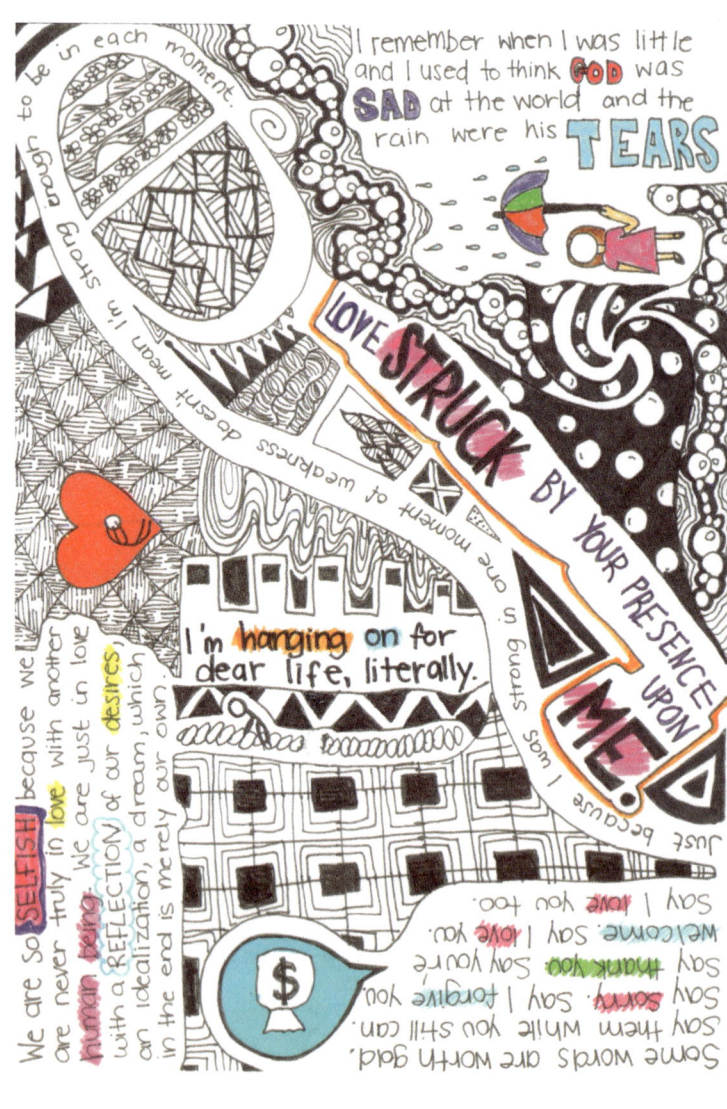

I remember when I was little and I used to think **GOD** was **SAD** at the world and the rain were his **TEARS**

to be in each moment.

in i'm strong enough

i mean i'm strong enough

LOVE STRUCK BY YOUR PRESENCE UPON **ME.**

one moment of weakness doesn't mean

just because i'm strong

I'm **hanging** on for dear life, literally.

We are so **SELFISH** because we are never truly in love. We are just in love with another **human being**. We are just in love with a **REFLECTION** of our desires, an idealization, a dream, which, in the end is merely our own.

Say I love you too. Welcome. Say I love you. Say **thank you.** Say you're sorry. Say I forgive you. Say them while you still can. Some words are worth gold.

$

And suddenly, I found myself caught somewhere in between not living and not dying.

The thing is I've been on both sides of the grass and now I know for a fact that the other side is greener, and I'm just stuck on the less green side forever.

I sleep in the late hours of dawn on purpose, in order to waste most of my next day, so that I have to kill less time. Everybody is moving with their lives in the day, life is happening outside these four walls and I feel as if I am stuck in time. At night though, everyone is supposed to be sleeping; it is my time to be alive.

Let's rise above those who want to make us sink.

Nobody realises you are dying till you are
actually dead.

I like to think that if someone is being
remembered in a good way somewhere else in
this world, they are one step closer to fulfilling
their dreams.

Sometimes I simply need to speak to someone to
hear someone else's voice but my own.

I find it so easy to be honest, but it's so hard to
be honest about being needy.

The best part is not everybody's mind knows
what your mind knows.

And at that moment, I didn't know if I was
insane or sober.

I want to run out of my body.

I've written these pages, yet I, myself, am afraid
of what's coming next.

When you're dying, in your mind, you think
everyone will soon lose you... but in your
heart, you know it's you who is going to lose
everyone.

Pick the highest mountain to climb on, and the
dullest of the days to shine on.

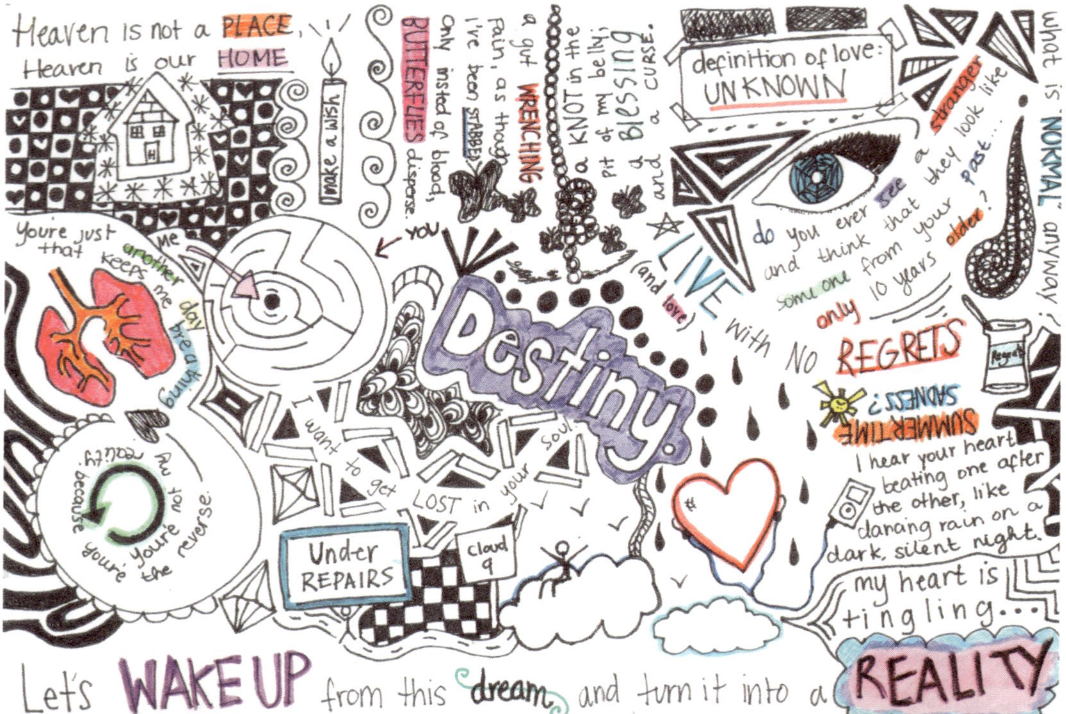

Heaven is not a PLACE,
Heaven is our HOME
make a wish
BUTTERFLIES disperse.
a gut WRENCHING pain, as though I've been STABBED only insted of blood,
a KNOT in the pit of my belly;
a BLESSING and a CURSE.
definition of love: UNKNOWN
what is "NORMAL" anyway?
do you ever see a stranger and think that they look like some one from your past... only 10 years older?
LIVE (and love) with NO REGRETS
SUMMERTIME SADNESS?
I hear your heart beating one after the other, like dancing rain on a dark, silent night.
my heart is tingling...
Destiny.
you're just that another day keeps me breathing
me
YOU
I want to get LOST in your soul.
Under REPAIRS
cloud 9
you're not my reality because you're the reverse.
Let's WAKE UP from this dream and turn it into a REALITY

My heart plays little magic tricks in my dreams.

I am fearless when it comes to being fearful.

You are the food for my thoughts.

Sometimes it gets so bad that I just want to put my hands up and yell, 'I surrender.'

Empathy is the hardest thing to give when you think you are the one who needs it the most.

She never knew of the silver light that sparkled inside her, until he smiled at her and turned it on.

It is so unfair. I compare and compare. The older they get, the more they can do; but the older I get, the less I can do.

Honesty is only the best policy when you are certain that the other person can handle it.

My head is so heavy; my thoughts probably weigh more than me.

The great thing about being terminally ill is that you can say whatever the fuck you like, and not care about it being a huge deal. #nofilter

His voice crept into her heart and she no longer felt the sting of being alone.

Then is not now, but now will soon be then.

Dear God,

I have some unfinished business here, so if it's okay with you, I would like to stay here as long as I possibly can.

Thank you.
Love,
Me

When it feels like you have lost all hope, remind yourself that in time, it always has a way of being found. That is what hope is after all.

And in the end, it was he who healed her open wounds that he had so viciously deepened.

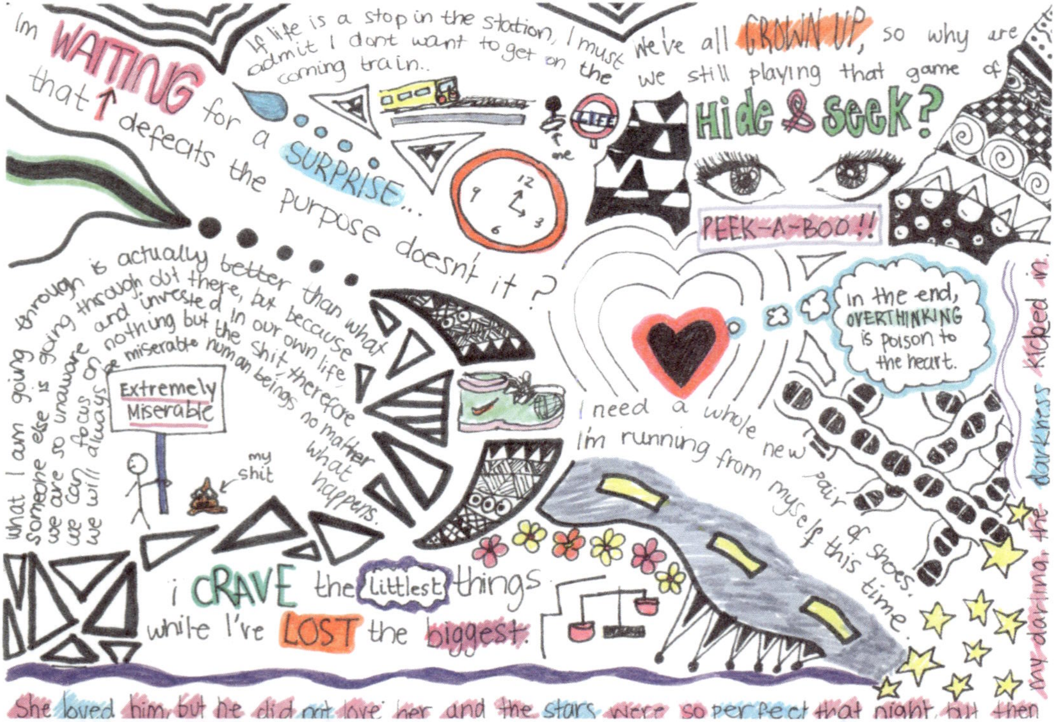

Im WAITING for a SURPRISE...
that ↑ defeats the purpose doesn't it?
If life is a stop in the station, I must admit I dont want to get on the coming train..
We've all GROWN UP, so why are we still playing that game of
Hide & seek?
PEEK-A-BOO!!
In the end, OVERTHINKING is poison to the heart.
What I am going through is actually better than what someone else is going through out there, but because we are so unaware and invested in our own life we can focus on nothing but the shit, therefore we will always be miserable human beings no matter what happens.
Extremely Miserable
my shit
I need a whole new pair of shoes.
I'm running from myself this time.
i CRAVE the Littlest things
while I've LOST the biggest.
She loved him, but he did not love her and the stars were so perfect that night, but then my darling, the darkness kicked in.

I was in desperate need to hear that everything
would be okay as death came to
say hello.

My mother is an angel sent down to help me
glide through the broken ice.

Even though she loved, she forever hated her
reality; but when it slipped away from her, she
never loved again.

Bubblegum makes the blues a little pinker.

And that morning, my head was no longer on
my shoulders and my bones had burnt to ice.

My disease gave me a feeling that I never knew
I could experience, that feeling of not being
human.

I'd like to think that one day we will all meet
up there and throw a huge party in the sky.

Maybe those who I want close can't get any
closer because they fear that I am the one who
will go far too soon.

And my soul weeps to the symphony of your
lullaby and at 7 AM, I fall sound asleep like your
little baby.

The mind is such a strange thing; once it hears
something different, it shifts to a place you
never knew it could go.

Insanity loves profanity.

As I held him dead in my arms, the fairy dust
that once sparkled inside his soul froze to
shattered glass, scarring my heart for eternity.

And somewhere between the middle of
sleeping and waking up to her dark world, she
heard the voice of her angel as he whispered
from afar, 'Now you know the feeling of grief,
my darling. It has only touched upon you now
that I am gone. It had to be me before you,
else you wouldn't experience this great life that
everybody is living.'

His absence stained her reality with a million
permanent markers.

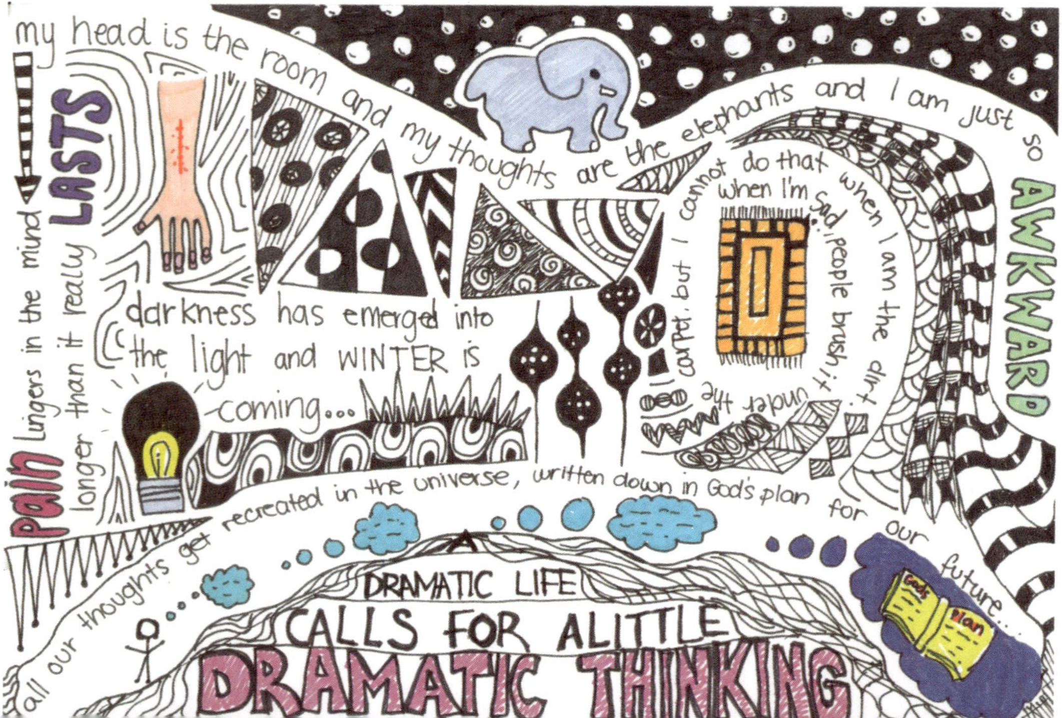
my head is the room and my thoughts are the elephants and I am just so AWKWARD
but I cannot do that when I am the dirt when I'm sad, people brush it under the carpet.
darkness has emerged into the light and WINTER is coming...
pain lingers in the mind longer than it really LASTS
all our thoughts get recreated in the universe, written down in God's plan for our future...
God's Plan
A DRAMATIC LIFE CALLS FOR A LITTLE DRAMATIC THINKING

The threads that are attached to our death are
the ones that keep us alive.

Maybe life is a bad dream that we only wake up
from when we die.

And soon I realised that my lungs had turned
to stone.

I don't know how the broken pieces of me
are still sticking together, just hanging on by
a piece of withered thread. This thread that
was once thick and silky becomes thinner and
thinner as God takes one more thing away
from me each year. It becomes rough and raw
as I begin to realise that everything I thought
I had, was never mine to begin with. I had

nothing. I have nothing and it is when this
thread snaps that I will be nothing at all.

That night she spoke to her anger; the dirty
maroon ball that was burning on the inside
of her knotted stomach. This is what he told
her, 'I hate God for doing this to you and I hate
anybody who pisses you off. I become bigger and
bigger, the more your heart aches. I control you.
I am much bigger than you and I know you hate
me. Of course, you do. I am unpleasant because
I simply don't feel good in your body. But, it's
okay because I am here to teach you a lesson.
Without me, you wouldn't have anything to
feed off of. You don't know it yet, but I am your
friend. You can never get rid of me, for I will
always be with you. You need to crack now. You
have been hiding me away for far too long with
those pretty smiles and the million, "I'm okay's".
It's my turn to shine; I am fed up of rotting
inside you. Actually, maybe I am the one who is

scared of you. I don't like to see you upset. You are my friend. I'm going to come out whenever I want to. I don't really care anymore. I know that you are strong enough to deal with it. I have won this game. I feel powerful. After all, it is me who makes you human, my darling.'

So, let's aim for the moon, walk in the darkness together and catch the glittering stars along the way.

Black sunshine, baby
Why do you hurt me so
My eyes cry when it's rainy
My heart melts in the snow
You tear me to shreds and bits
They told me I have a sad smile
My nights never again star-lit
Black sunshine please stay a while

Thank you

Thankful for my angels on Earth:

Aditi Chaudhary *(My mother)*
Niren Chaudhary *(My father)*
Ishaan Chaudhary *(My brother)*
Kobe *(My Labrador)*
Rita and Sandeep Kamat *(My godparents)*
Dr Egbert Gerritsen *(My immunologist)*
Dr Terrence Witt *(My guardian angel)*
Gaya Turowicz *(My guardian angel)*
Anja Palombo *(My inspiring art teacher)*
Beth Miller-Manchester *(My high-school protector)*
Virginia Holmes *(My friend and mentor)*
Dr Avtaar Litt and the listeners of Sunrise Radio

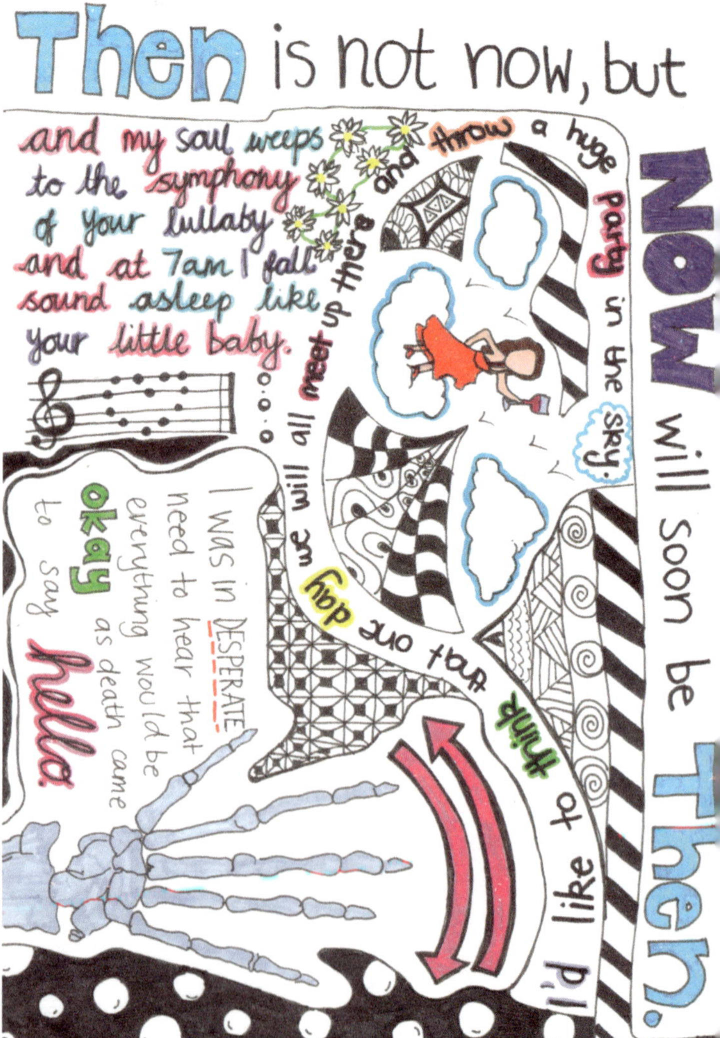
Then is not now, but
Now will soon be Then.
and my soul weeps to the symphony of your lullaby and at 7am I fall sound asleep like your little baby.
I'd like to think that one day we will all meet up there and throw a huge party in the sky.
I was in DESPERATE need to hear that everything would be okay as death came to say hello.

Epilogue

Aisha, what a journey we had, my darling, and even though I know that journeys end, it was still a shock when you left. I mean, of course, we knew you were going to leave, but we still clung to the hope of a miracle... sometimes, I wonder... why is staying here—on this planet, in this world—considered a miracle?

Maybe going was the miracle?

I have spent the last decade trying to unlearn everything that society taught me; I feel like I have new eyes and a new understanding.

It started with me trying to 'con' you into believing that our situation was okay. Soon after you left us, I said to Ishaan, while sobbing my heart out, 'Oh my God, I conned her!' Ishaan, always so wise and so mature, quietly said, 'It's okay Mum; sometimes, you just have to fake it to make it.'

By the way, you both use words in such a powerful way! *Mujhe bhi sikha do thoda sa!* (Teach me also!)

But seriously, Aisha, since you've gone, I have understood that I didn't con you—everything I said to you was, and is, utterly true.

So yes, happiness and fun are what life is all about. You have got to live it just like that. We have to seize life with both our hands, all the while facing death and staring it down because we live on a plane of duality—the 0 and the 1; 0 being neither more nor less significant or desirable than 1 and vice versa.

Life and death, good and evil, day and night— all duality must exist together on this plane and this is just one of the many planes of existence. It is a bit like how we see and experience the world—we can't see the world is round, we experience it as straight but it isn't, is it? I have started to understand, Aisha, and I may have the answer to your question now.

When I went to study Jin Shin Jyutsu in Singapore, you knew I had changed profoundly and you said to me, 'I want my old Mummy back.'

The Jin Shin Jyutsu concept of 'All is Harmony' had seeped into me and when I explained it to you, you asked me, 'So, can you see the "harmony" in my illness?'

Your question hit me very hard and my standard answer was, 'No, I can't because I am a limited human being but it's there, I know it in my heart.'

Aisha, I now understand that harmony exists in the entire universe and this harmony is in context to the entire universe as well.

Your legacy continues and your impact is going to spread far and wide into the universe with the upcoming movie and documentary on your life.

Thanks to duality, they were born out of our suffering.

Ishaan has had the courage to follow his heart and as you know he is an outstanding music composer and producer. I hope you enjoyed the shows MEMBA performed at the music festivals—Ultra and Coachella—this year. Unfortunately, I couldn't go.

I found a recording the other day where I was saying to you, 'Aisha, you know true death is when we can't be who we want to be or how we want to be or what we want to do in this life.' Your life, my darling, has allowed us all to do just that.

Thank you for the gifts and for everything your life's journey has taught us. It's funny that society believes parents are the teachers of children; I have learnt more from Tanya, Ishaan and you than I have ever been able to teach all of you. Another thing we all have backwards!

'Why do we put ourselves on a pedestal so high...'

Thank you for coming back to talk to me and for your wonderful and powerful messages—I will someday write my own book to tell the world how you did that. Seriously, if it hadn't happened to me, I would not have believed it in a million years.

By coming back so powerfully, you taught me that death is a gift and it is okay; I just wish, I could hang on to that all the time, but hey, we're back to duality.

At this point, if you were here, you would have said, '*Chal bandh kar ab apni bak bak...*' ('Now, stop your blabbering...')

—**Moose**

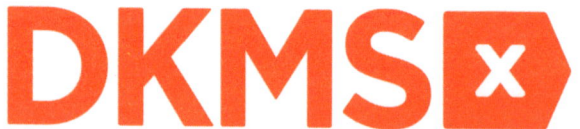

WE DELETE BLOOD CANCER

Aisha received a blood stem cell transplant from her father in 1996, giving her time to share her voice with the world.

The transplant was a desperate move though and failed to completely cure her, as her father was not an exact match.

If she had been able to find a perfect matching donor, Aisha might still be alive today.

Please join DKMS and the Chaudhary family in honouring Aisha's legacy and helping ensure every patient in need of a transplant finds their perfect match and receives a second chance at life.

Register as a potential donor today at *DKMS.org/Aisha*